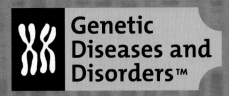

Genetic Diseases and Disorders™

Hemophilia

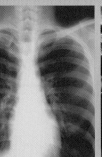
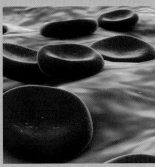
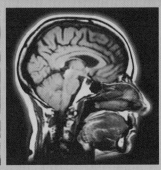
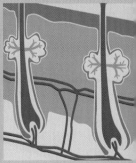

Jeri Freedman

The Rosen Publishing Group, Inc., New York

To my niece and nephew, Laura and Matthew Freedman

Published in 2007 by The Rosen Publishing Group, Inc.

29 East 21st Street, New York, NY 10010

Library of Congress Cataloging-in-Publication Data

Freedman, Jeri.
Hemophilia / Jeri Freedman.
    p. cm.—(Genetic diseases and disorders)
Includes bibliographical references and index.
ISBN 1-4042-0698-1 (lib. bdg.)
1. Hemophilia.
I. Title. II. Series.
RC642.F37 2007
616.1'572—dc22

2005030124

Manufactured in the United States of America

On the cover: Foreground: Illustration of red blood cells. Background: Fibrin network on a fresh wound during the formation of a blood clot.

Contents

Introduction

We have all cut ourselves at one time or another. When that happens, the blood clots, stopping the flow of blood from the injury. When someone has hemophilia, however, his or her blood doesn't clot normally. It can take a long time to stop the flow of blood. Injuries that are not normally serious for most people can be life-threatening for people who suffer from hemophilia.

Hemophilia is a genetic disease. It is caused by a defect, or mistake, in one of a person's genes. Genes are the elements in our cells that carry the information that determines what traits we have, such as hair or eye color. In the case of hemophilia, there is a defect in the gene that controls the production of one of the substances that causes blood to clot. This defect can be passed on from parents to their children.

What is it like to have hemophilia? Let's take Alex as an example. Much of the time, Alex does the same things everyone else does. He goes to school, likes to swim, and works part-time at a grocery store. Unlike other people, however, Alex must always be alert for cuts and bruises on his body. When he notices that he is bleeding, he needs to take care of the injury immediately. On his own or sometimes with help, he mixes the medicine he needs for treatment and takes care of the bleeding. Sometimes other students at school pick on him because he's different. And sometimes he feels angry and frustrated that he has to deal with all this extra stuff that other people don't. However, Alex knows that he's not alone. Presently, about 20,000 Americans and 3,800 Canadians are living with the disease. The World Federation of Hemophilia estimates that there are more than 500,000 people worldwide with hemophilia.

This book begins by examining the nature and history of hemophilia. It then discusses the symptoms of and treatments for the disease. Finally, it takes a look at some of the recent research aimed at discovering better ways to treat the disease, with the long-term goal of finding a cure.

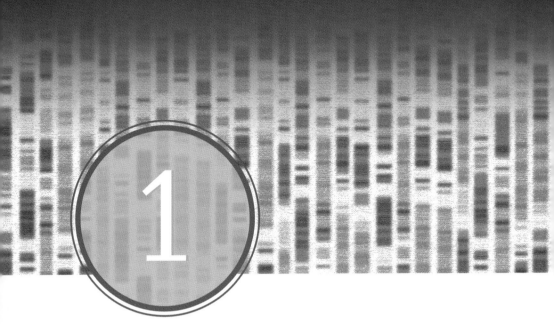

The Bleeding Disease

Hemophilia is caused by a problem with one of the substances in the blood that makes it clot. Blood clotting is a sequence of chemical activities. When a wound occurs in a blood vessel, blood cells called platelets clump together to start plugging the hole. This process is referred to as platelet adhesion. The first platelets to arrive at the damaged area put out chemicals that attract proteins called clotting factors. When the clotting factors arrive on the scene, they assist in the formation of a chain of proteins called fibrin. The strands of fibrin form a net of tough fibers around the platelets, holding them firmly in place. When someone has hemophilia, one of the clotting factors is missing or doesn't work properly. The blood clot that

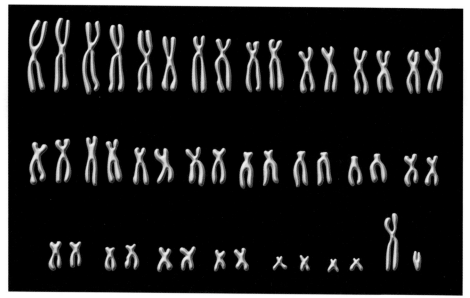

Human beings have twenty-three pairs of chromosomes, for a total of forty-six. Each pair consists of one chromosome from each parent. Pictured above is a complete set of male chromosomes. Defects on the X chromosome (second from right on the bottom row) can lead to a lack of clotting factor VIII or IX, resulting in hemophilia.

forms is soft and can easily fall apart. This makes it difficult to stop the bleeding.

Genetics and DNA

Genetic information is transmitted from parents to offspring via chromosomes found in the nuclei (central core) of cells. Chromosomes are structures made up of protein and deoxyribonucleic acid (DNA). Genes are sequences of DNA located at specific places on a chromosome. Genes act as blueprints for the production of proteins, which are the main substances that make up our bodies. A gene or combination of genes code for a specific trait, such as eye color or a clotting factor.

Almost every cell in your body contains two copies of each chromosome. One of the copies comes from your mother, and one comes from your father. Sperm and egg cells, however, contain only one copy of each chromosome. Sperm and egg cells are formed by a process called meiosis. In this process, the pairs of chromosomes are copied then line up at different ends of the cell's nucleus. The cell then divides twice to form four cells. In this way, sperm and egg cells are formed that each contain one-half of each chromosome pair. The sperm and egg cells later join, and an embryo is formed. The embryo receives one-half of each pair of its chromosomes from its mother and one-half from its father.

Sometimes one of the genes that makes up a chromosome has an error in its sequence, which causes it to work incorrectly or not at all. In the case of hemophilia, this can result in the body not producing one of the clotting factors. This type of error in a gene is usually inherited from a parent who already has the mistake. Sometimes, though, the change is a mutation, or spontaneous change, that occurs when the chromosomes are copied during meiosis or early development of the embryo. Scientists estimate that about two-thirds of all new cases of hemophilia are the result of an inherited genetic defect. The other one-third come from new mutations in a gene.

Who Gets Hemophilia?

Hemophilia is much more common in boys than in girls. This is because the gene for hemophilia is located on the X chromosome, which is one of the chromosomes that determines the

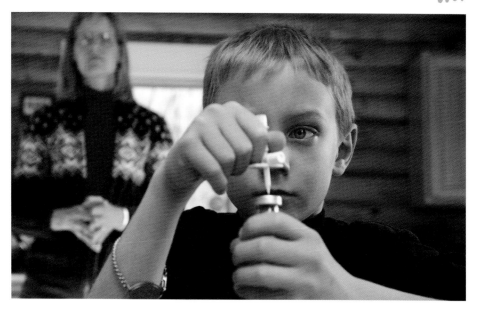

Many children with hemophilia take medicine every week to prevent bleeding problems. It is important for children to learn how to prepare their medication, so they can take it by themselves if needed. Hemophilia medication can cost as much as $1,000 per dose.

sex of a baby. Females have two X chromosomes. Males have one X chromosome and one Y chromosome. Children get an X chromosome from their mother and an X or Y chromosome from their father. The gene for hemophilia is what is known as an X-linked recessive gene. Since a male has only one X chromosome, if his X chromosome contains a defective gene for one of the clotting factors, he will have hemophilia. In contrast, even if a female gets an X chromosome from one parent that contains a defective gene for one of the clotting factors, if she gets a healthy gene for that factor on the X chromosome she receives from the other parent, she will not get hemophilia.

A female with one normal X chromosome and one X chromosome containing the defective gene is called a

TCGATTCTGAACATGATACGTACTGGTCCACTAGAACTGAACTCGAGAGGTACTA

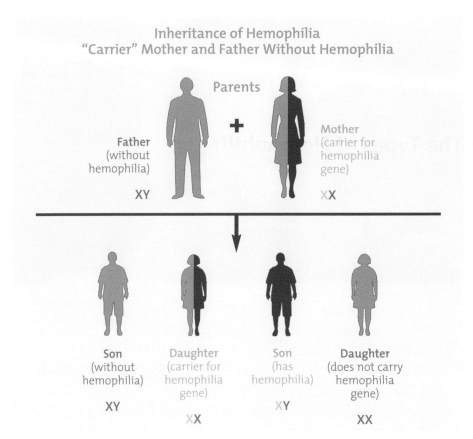

Inheritance of Hemophilia
"Carrier" Mother and Father Without Hemophilia

Parents

Father
(without
hemophilia)

XY

Mother
(carrier for
hemophilia
gene)

XX

Son
(without
hemophilia)

XY

Daughter
(carrier for
hemophilia
gene)

XX

Son
(has
hemophilia)

XY

Daughter
(does not carry
hemophilia
gene)

XX

A mother who has the gene for hemophilia on one of her X chromosomes can pass the gene on to her children. If she has a son, the son has a 50 percent chance of having hemophilia. If she has a daughter, the daughter has a 50 percent chance of being a carrier of the disease.

carrier. Carriers of hemophilia sometimes have other bleeding-related problems, even though they do not have hemophilia. They may bleed more than normal from menstruation, surgery, or nosebleeds. Each time a carrier becomes pregnant, her child has a 50 percent chance of inheriting the defective gene. Any of her sons who receive the defective gene will have hemophilia. Her daughters will not have the disease if they get a normal gene from their father. A female can only have hemophilia if she inherits defective genes from both her mother and father. This is extremely rare.

The Types of Hemophilia

Blood clotting requires more than a dozen different clotting factors. There are several different types of hemophilia. Each type is caused by the lack of a specific factor.

- Type A is caused by a lack of factor VIII. This is the most common type of hemophilia, affecting 85 percent of those with the disease. It is also called classic hemophilia.
- Type B is caused by a lack of factor IX. Hemophilia type B is sometimes called Christmas disease, after Stephen Christmas, a Canadian who was the first person diagnosed with this disorder, in 1952.
- About 1 percent of all cases of hemophilia are caused by problems with factors V, VII, X, XI, or XIII.

Hemophilia can be mild, moderate, or severe, depending on the amount of blood-clotting factor a patient produces. People with as little as 10 percent of the normal level of clotting factor may only have serious bleeding problems after medical procedures such as surgery or after a severe injury. Excessive bleeding after these events may be the first sign that someone has hemophilia.

Severe hemophilia occurs when a person has less than 1 percent of the normal level of clotting factor. In these cases, spontaneous bleeding (bleeding that occurs for no identifiable reason) can result from the ordinary wear and tear of everyday activities. Those suffering from severe hemophilia can

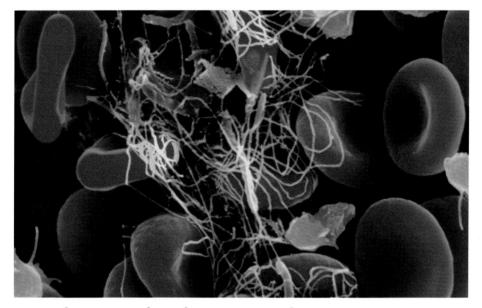

Researchers use tools such as scanning electron microscopes to study events in the body too small to see with the naked eye. This micrograph (picture taken through a microscope) shows the strands of fibrin *(yellow)* surrounding red blood cells and platelets *(blue)*. Clotting factors link strands of fibrin to form a tough "mesh" that holds platelets together to form a hemostatic (blood-stopping) plug.

suffer spontaneous bleeding several times a month if they do not undergo preventive treatment.

Another disorder, von Willebrand's disease, is closely related to hemophilia. This disease is named after the Finnish doctor who discovered it in the 1920s. In von Willebrand's disease, a clotting factor known as the von Willebrand factor is defective. Although the blood of someone with von Willebrand's disease will clot, it takes an abnormally long time to do so. This disease is 100 times more common than hemophilia. Unlike hemophilia, it is not linked to the X chromosome and affects both men and women equally.

Where Are Clotting Factors Made?

Factor VIII is produced primarily by cells in the liver, although some is also made by cells in the kidney, lymphatic (immune) system, and other locations. Normally, factor VIII lasts for about twelve hours before being broken down in the body. Von Willebrand factor circulates in the blood along with factor VIII to keep it from breaking down too soon. Von Willebrand factor also helps concentrate factor VIII at sites where damage has occurred. Factor IX, which is defective in hemophilia type B, is also made in the liver. It requires vitamin K to function and lasts about twenty-four hours in the body.

Hemophilia in History

Abu al-Qasim al-Zahrawi, also known as Albucasis, was a famous Muslim doctor born in the tenth century in Córdoba, Spain. He invented a number of surgical instruments, wrote a thirty-volume medical encyclopedia, and was thought by many to be the most important physician in the Middle Ages. One entry in his encyclopedia described a family in which the men died of prolonged bleeding from minor wounds. This is believed to be the first detailed description of hemophilia ever recorded.

The first modern description of the disease was made by Dr. G. W. C. Consbruch of Germany in 1793. A few years later, scientific investigation into the disease was stimulated by John Conrad Otto, a doctor living in Philadelphia, Pennsylvania. He published an

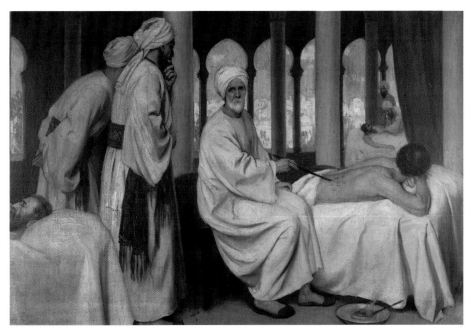

Abu al-Qasim al-Zahrawi is depicted healing a patient in this painting from the early twentieth century. Much of the medical knowledge of the ancient Greeks was preserved and expanded on by Arab physicians such as al-Zahrawi during the Middle Ages. Al-Zahrawi's medical books were translated into Latin in the twelfth century and became the standard medical reference on a wide range of diseases.

article in 1803 entitled "An Account of an Haemorrhagic Disposition Existing in Certain Families." "Haemorrhage" means to bleed uncontrollably (although today it is usually spelled "hemorrhage"). In this article, Otto traced the inheritance of hemophilia back through three generations of a family. He demonstrated that the disorder afflicted men in multiple generations, indicating that there was a genetic link.

The term "hemophilia" was used in print for the first time in 1828 by Friedrich Hopff, a medical student at the University of Zurich in Switzerland. He wrote a paper entitled "Uber die Haemophilie oder die erbliche Anlage zu

HEMOPHILIA IN ANCIENT TIMES

Near AD 100, Rabbi Judah the Patriarch stated that baby boys did not have to undergo circumcision (removal of the foreskin of the penis) if they had a brother who had died of bleeding after this procedure. One thousand years later this ruling was extended by Moses Maimonides, a rabbi and lawmaker who lived in Egypt. He stated that if a woman married a second time, her sons by this second marriage should also be exempt from circumcision if any of her sons by her first marriage had suffered bleeding problems as a result of the procedure. These rulings showed that even far back in time people had a sense that certain disorders could be inherited, even if they did not understand exactly how the process worked.

todlichen Blutungen." The title translates from German as "On Hemophilia or Hereditary Fatal Bleeding." This work described inherited bleeding disorders that only affected men. He noted that the disease was passed on by women who didn't suffer from the disease themselves. From that time on, "hemophilia" was used to refer to the disease. The word combines the Latin terms *hem*, which means "blood," and *philia*, which means "love" or "attraction." In other words, hemophilia literally means "love of blood."

 ## The Royal Disease

Not all hemophilia is inherited. Sometimes it occurs as the result of a random mutation, or change, in a gene. That is

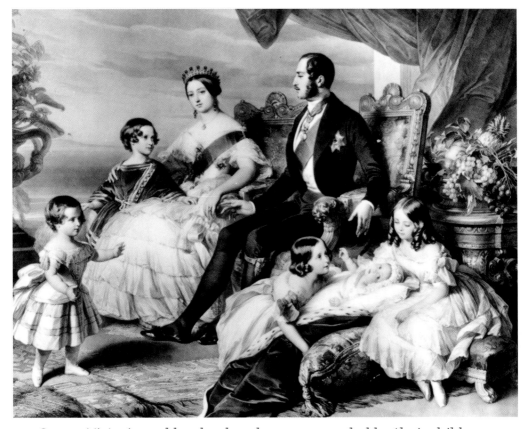

Queen Victoria and her husband are surrounded by their children in this painting from 1848. From left to right, Prince Alfred (wearing a dress), Prince Edward, Queen Victoria, Prince Albert, Princess Alice, Princess Helena, and Princess Victoria. Both Queen Victoria and Princess Alice were carriers of the hemophilia gene.

what happened in the case of the English royal family. Queen Victoria came to the throne of England in 1837. At that time, there was no history of hemophilia in her family. However, in 1853, Queen Victoria gave birth to her eighth child, Leopold, and he had hemophilia. Since there was no history of hemophilia in Victoria's family, a spontaneous change must have

CGATTCTGAACATGATACGTACTGGTCCACTAGAACTGAACTCGAGAGGTACIA

occurred in the gene that came from the queen. According to an article that appeared in 1868 in the *British Medical Journal*, Leopold often had serious bleeding problems. In 1884, Leopold suffered bleeding in his brain after a fall and died at the age of thirty-one.

Over time, hemophilia would spread from Queen Victoria's family into the other royal families of Europe. Because of this it was known as the "royal disease." Two of Queen Victoria's daughters, Alice and Beatrice, were carriers of the hemophilia gene. Beatrice had two sons with hemophilia and one who did not. She also had a daughter, Eugenia, who was a carrier. In 1906, Eugenia married King Alfonso of Spain. Their eldest son, Alfonso, and youngest son, Gonzalo, both had hemophilia. In the 1930s, they both died of wounds received in auto accidents, complicated by their hemophilia.

Queen Victoria's daughter Alice married Prince Henry of Prussia, part of modern-day Germany. The prince was her first cousin, and their two sons Waldemar and Henry both had hemophilia. Waldemar bled to death at age four. His brother Henry lived until age fifty-six.

A Sick Child and the Mad Monk

In the early twentieth century, Russia was ruled by Czar Nicholas II. One of Queen Victoria of England's granddaughters, Alix (called Alexandra in Russia), married Nicholas. In 1904, Alexandra gave birth to a son, Alexis, who had hemophilia. This event would have a major impact on the course of Russian history.

At that time, there were very few ways to treat hemophilia and Alexis suffered from debilitating pain. A Russian monk named Gregory Efimovich Rasputin seemed to have the ability

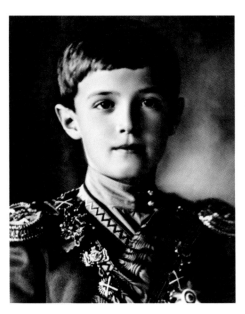

Alexis, son of Czar Nicholas II, suffered great pain from bleeding into his joints because of his hemophilia. He inherited the disease from his mother, Alexandra, a granddaughter of Queen Victoria of England. Because of Alexis's illness, his mother devoted herself almost entirely to his welfare.

to ease Alexis's suffering. Alexandra made the monk a member of the royal household. In time, Rasputin came to have great influence over the royal family.

Rasputin was popular with many of the ordinary people in Russia. They saw Rasputin as one of their own who had made good. The aristocrats, however, feared that his influence over the royal family was greater than their own. They expressed their distrust of the monk to the royal family. Alexandra refused to have him sent away, however, because he helped her son.

In June 1914, World War I struck Europe, and Russia became involved. Many powerful people began to turn against Czar Nicholas. They felt that many of his decisions were endangering Russia. But the aristocrats didn't solely place the blame on the czar. The aristocrats felt that Czar Nicholas was allowing Rasputin to influence his decisions in order to keep the monk in his household where he could help his son. For example, Nicholas allowed Rasputin to

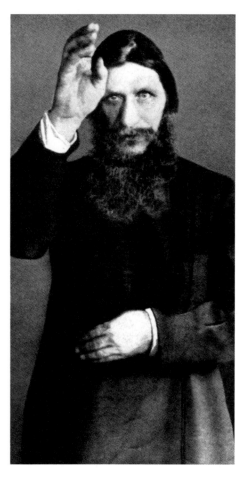

The monk Rasputin was initially a spiritual advisor to the Russian royal family. His ability to ease the suffering of Alexis allowed him to gain vast influence over the royal family. Eventually, he was able to exert his power to affect political decisions made by Czar Nicholas and Alexandra.

decide which government ministers to hire and fire. On December 30, 1916, the aristocrats lured Rasputin into a trap and killed him. This angered the common Russian people, who felt he had represented their viewpoint to the royal family. Within a few months of Rasputin's murder, the Russian Social Democratic Workers' Party, also called the Bolsheviks, seized power in Russia. They imprisoned and then, in July 1918, executed Czar Nicholas and his entire family. Many historians feel that Rasputin's presence and death were two of the underlying causes of the revolution. Thus, Alexis's hemophilia helped change the course of life in Russia.

Living with Hemophilia

The major symptom of hemophilia is uncontrolled bleeding. Sometimes the bleeding is obvious, as in the case of a nosebleed. Sometimes, however, bleeding occurs in the joints or the head and cannot be seen externally. Signs of internal bleeding include a tingling feeling and warmth and stiffness in the area involved. If not treated promptly, internal bleeding can cause serious damage to the body's joints, muscles, and organs.

A painful headache, drowsiness, or confusion can indicate bleeding in the head. Bleeding in the head is especially dangerous because it can cause brain damage and even death if it is not quickly discovered and stopped. It is not the bleeding from external wounds that is dangerous to those

CGATTCTGAACATGATACGTACTGGTCCACTAGAACTGAACTCGAGAGGTACTA

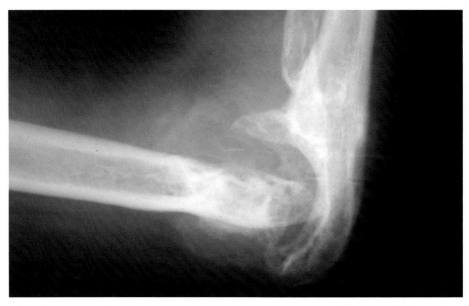

Bleeding into the joints is a common symptom of hemophilia. This type of bleeding often occurs in the knee and elbow joints. Here you can see the bulge where bleeding into the elbow joint has caused the tissue to swell. This bleeding is painful and can damage the bones and tissue in the joints.

with hemophilia. Such external bleeding can usually be controlled by first aid.

Diagnosis of Hemophilia

Many of the symptoms seen in hemophilia can also occur in other types of diseases. Therefore, if hemophilia is suspected, the doctor has to perform various tests to make sure that it is definitely the cause of the patient's symptoms. If the doctor thinks a patient might have hemophilia, he or she does a complete physical exam. The exam includes getting the

SIGNS OF HEMOPHILIA

- Very large bruises resulting from small accidents that would produce only a small bruise on a healthy person
- Frequent bleeding from gums, mouth, or nose
- Bleeding in urine or stool
- Joint pain and damage as a result of bleeding in a joint
- Muscle pain as a result of bleeding in muscle tissue that causes pressure on nearby nerves

patient's medical history to see, among other things, if the patient's parents had hemophilia. In addition, the doctor does several tests. One of these tests is called a complete blood count (CBC). It measures how many red blood cells are in the patient's blood. A low number of red blood cells may be a sign of excessive bleeding. Other blood tests include checking for the presence of specific blood-clotting factors, DNA testing to see if the patient has a defective gene, and a test that measures how long it takes a patient's blood to clot.

Playing It Safe

From a very early age, people with hemophilia must take special measures to minimize bleeding. For instance, when a child is learning to walk, it may be necessary for him or her to wear padded clothing to avoid injuries from falling or bumping into things. A child with hemophilia may have to avoid contact sports for the same reason. When undergoing surgery or dental procedures, people with hemophilia may need to receive an infusion of clotting factors (a solution introduced into the body through a needle inserted into a vein). This is done so that they don't bleed uncontrollably and will heal better. Hemophiliacs also need to avoid certain medications that contain aspirin or other compounds that can lead to increased bleeding. If serious bleeding does occur, a person with hemophilia may need to receive transfusions of blood.

Treating Hemophilia

The first approach to treating hemophilia was simply to replace the blood lost with a blood transfusion. In a transfusion, blood flows down a tube into the patient's body through a needle placed in a vein. Transfusion with whole blood (blood that has not been separated into liquid and solid parts) introduces blood-clotting factors that are missing in the hemophiliac's own blood. The first successful treatment of hemophilia by blood transfusion was performed in 1840 by the English physician Samuel Lane.

In 1934, another way to treat hemophilia was discovered by R. G. Macfarlane, also an English physician. He found that venom from a snake called a Russell's viper could be used to increase blood clotting in a patient with hemophilia. Under the name Stypen, a commercial version of the venom was produced.

In 1936, plasma was first used to treat hemophilia. Plasma is the clear, yellowish fluid that is left after the solid blood cells have been removed. It contains elements that cause blood to clot, such as fibrin, but, because the solid blood cells have been removed, is less likely to cause bad reactions.

As late as the 1950s and 1960s, people suffering from hemophilia were treated with transfusions of whole blood or

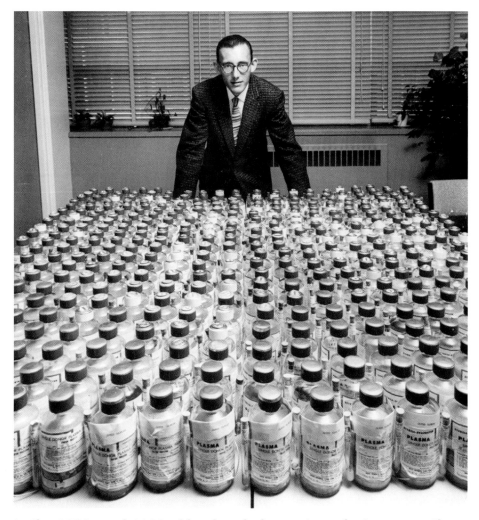

In the 1950s and 1960s, blood and plasma transfusions were the primary method of treating hemophilia. This photo shows one man with hemophilia who had to have daily transfusions of plasma. He is shown with the 365 bottles representing transfusions for one year. One problem with relying on transfusions to treat hemophilia is that this type of treatment generally must be done in a hospital or clinic. Today, other treatments are available to treat hemophilia in addition to transfusion.

plasma. Unfortunately, the treatments were often unsuccessful because the transfused blood or plasma did not contain high enough concentrations of clotting factor to stop very serious internal bleeding. Today, however, a better understanding of the disease has resulted in the production of medications and treatments that make it possible for most people with hemophilia to live a normal lifespan.

Clotting-Factor Infusions

A common treatment today is for people with hemophilia to receive infusions of clotting factor on a regular basis. This provides protection against uncontrolled bleeding in the event that an injury occurs. However, clotting-factor infusions are not always successful. One of the problems of receiving an infusion is the development of immunity to the factors. This happens because our immune system is designed to seek out and neutralize foreign particles that get into our bodies. Sometimes when external clotting factors are introduced into a person's blood, the immune system recognizes these elements as foreign particles. The immune system then produces proteins called antibodies. The antibodies attach to the clotting factors when they enter the bloodstream, marking them as invaders. Immune system cells then engulf and destroy the clotting factors.

Inhibitors

The antibodies that attach to the clotting factors are called inhibitors. They inhibit the action of the clotting factors and make it impossible for them to do their jobs. Most facilities that treat people with hemophilia test for inhibitors. It's also common

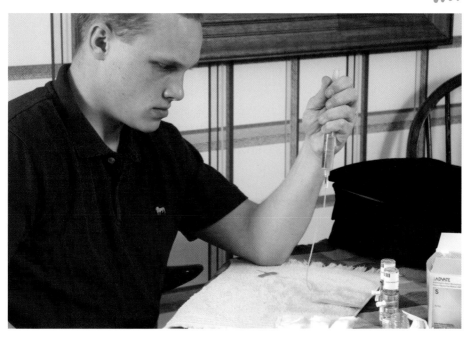

This patient is preparing tubing prior to infusing clotting factor. It is common for patients to learn to prepare clotting factor and infuse themselves. Therefore, they do not have to go to a medical facility for treatment, but can prepare the medication and treat themselves at home.

for their presence to be detected when a patient continues having bleeding problems despite treatment or when patients who previously showed improvement start to bleed again.

If the presence of an inhibitor is suspected, the patient is given a test called a Bethesda assay. The test measures the strength of the inhibitor. The strength of the inhibitor is called its "titer." The titer of inhibitors is measured in Bethesda units, or BUs. A high titer is five BUs or more. Someone with a low titer might respond to treatment with a larger infusion of clotting factor. Those who have a high titer, however, will simply put out more inhibitors to neutralize the clotting factors, and therefore must rely on other types of treatment.

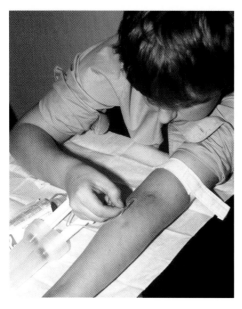

Youngsters with hemophilia can learn to infuse clotting factor themselves. The clotting factor comes in powdered form and is mixed with fluid such as saline (salt) solution. The solution is then administered through a tubing and needle set, which, in most cases, is provided with the clotting factor by the supplier.

Those most at risk for developing inhibitors include people of Hispanic or African American heritage and those who are younger than twenty years of age. Treatment options for those with inhibitors to human blood-clotting factors include the use of factors that have been altered in a laboratory, or factors that have been derived from pig rather than human blood. The problem with all of these treatments, however, is that they work in some people but not others. In some cases, they may also cause dangerous blood clots that block a blood vessel so that no blood can get through. Therefore, an appropriate treatment must be established for each patient on a case-by-case basis.

Prophylaxis

"Prophylaxis" means to take precautions before a problem starts, which may enable one to avoid the problem altogether.

In hemophilia, this term is applied to the regular infusion of clotting factors to prevent bleeding problems before they begin. Typically, people receive infusions of clotting factor two or three times per week. This helps them keep the level of factors VIII or IX in their blood high enough for clotting to occur. It is common for this treatment to begin when patients are young, often between two and four years old.

One problem with using prophylaxis to treat hemophilia is the need to give infusions of clotting factor several times a week. This requires locating a vein for the needle to enter every time the infusion must be given. This is an uncomfortable situation, especially for children.

An alternative is the use of a port-a-cath, or implantable venous access device (IVAD). This device is implanted under the skin either in the upper chest or under the patient's arm. It is left there for a year or more. The device consists of a long thin tube that is inserted into a large chest or arm vein, and a reservoir that holds the medication to be supplied. The medication is placed in the reservoir and goes through the tube and into the vein. The major drawback of such a device is that patients often develop infections where the device is implanted. Also, the tip of the catheter can become plugged with a blood clot. Still, many people prefer the device because it makes receiving the medication much easier than other methods.

Unlocking the Secrets
of Hemophilia

4

Since the twentieth century, scientific discoveries have significantly advanced the understanding and treatment of hemophilia. As mentioned earlier, in 1936, scientists discovered that plasma could be used to treat hemophilia. In 1937, two researchers at Harvard Medical School, A. J. Patek and F. H. L. Taylor, discovered an improved way to treat the disease. They discovered that solids removed from plasma, rather than whole plasma, could be injected to make blood clot faster. In 1939, Kenneth Brinkhous at the University of North Carolina demonstrated that people with hemophilia lack a component of the plasma, which he called antihemophilic factor. Today, this substance is known as factor VIII.

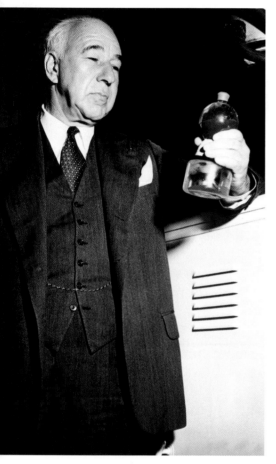

Dr. Edwin Cohn, director of the Harvard University Laboratory of Physical Chemistry, holds the original device used to separate blood into its various components. This is done by spinning the blood in this special bottle very rapidly in a machine called a centrifuge. The part of blood called plasma, a yellowish fluid, contains the clotting factors.

In 1944, a doctor in Buenos Aires, Argentina, named Alfredo Pavlovsky found in laboratory tests that blood from one patient with hemophilia could cause the blood of another hemophilia patient to clot. This meant that there were two different clotting factors in the blood (later identified as factors VIII and IX). A patient could lack one but have the other. The same year, an American biochemist at Harvard Medical School, Edwin Cohn, developed a technique for separating plasma into its component parts. This process, called fractionation, allowed Cohn and his colleagues to demonstrate that one of the blood fractions, named Cohn Fraction I, contained the blood-clotting factors. Armand Quick, an American doctor, reached the same conclusion that year. The work of these researchers laid the foundation for advances in understanding hemophilia for decades to come.

Advances in Treating Hemophilia

In 1955, three American pathologists, Kenneth Brinkhous, Robert Langdell, and Robert Wagner, developed the first method of giving patients infusions of factor VIII. Unfortunately, there were problems with this early form of treatment. In the 1950s, plasma from animals such as pigs and cows was used in hemophilia treatments, and many people had serious allergic reactions to these animal products.

In 1964, R. G. Macfarlane identified the process by which various factors work in series to clot blood. In this process, the factors line up like a series of dominoes—when the first one is knocked over, it affects the next, which affects the next, and so on. In the blood, this sequential activation of clotting factors is called the coagulation cascade. Scientists now better understood how blood clots were formed and began to search for new ways to treat hemophilia.

Frozen Factors

In the middle of the 1960s, Judith Pool, a doctor working at Stanford University, made a discovery that tremendously advanced hemophilia treatment. She discovered that slowly thawing frozen plasma resulted in the precipitation, or depositing, of solid material at the bottom of a container. Such deposits are called cryoprecipitates ("cryo" means frozen). Dr. Pool found that the cryoprecipitates were high in factor VIII. They had much greater power to make blood clot than whole plasma did.

Cryoprecipitates allowed the hemophilia patient to treat him- or herself from home instead of having to travel to a

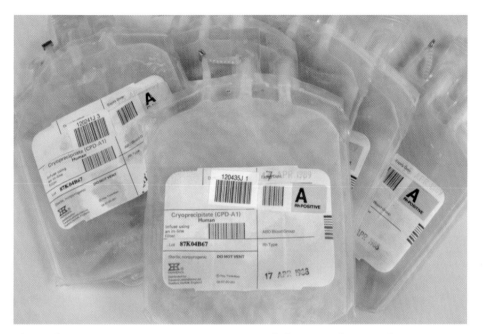

These bags contain cryoprecipitates of clotting factors for use in treating hemophilia. Blood is divided into four types (A, B, AB, and O). All people have one of these four blood types. Cryoprecipitates are matched to the specific blood type of the person receiving them. In this case, it is matched to type A.

hospital. The cryoprecipitate could be kept frozen at home, and if necessary, a local doctor could perform the infusion after thawing some of the patient's supply of the material. Following Dr. Pool's initial work, researchers at the Plasma Fractionation Laboratory (PFL) in Oxford, England, produced cryoprecipitates of various other important clotting factors, such as factors VII, XI, and XIII. By 1968, freeze-drying was found to be possible with the cryoprecipitates. This resulted in a powdered form of the clotting factor that could be kept at home and used as necessary.

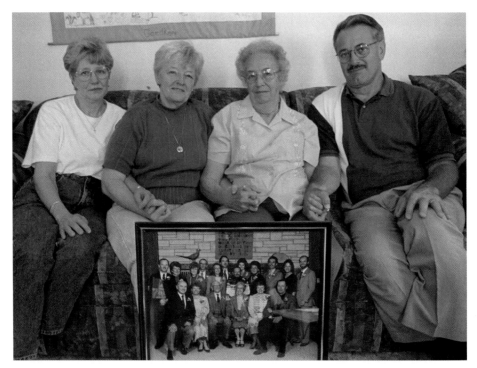

Four members of the Goedken family reflect on members of the family who died of AIDS (acquired immunodeficiency syndrome). In all, five brothers with hemophilia, two of the brothers' wives, and one of their children died. The brothers contracted the AIDS virus from using contaminated blood products. The virus then spread to other family members.

Dangers Lurking in the Blood Supply

However, the use of cryoprecipitates was not without drawbacks. The plasma from which the precipitates are made is the result of pooling a large quantity of plasma from thousands of individual donors. One problem with pooling blood from so many different people is that it increases the chance of contamination by a virus. Viruses present in plasma will be passed on to those who use the plasma or precipitates made from it. A few of the most serious viruses that can be passed on are hepatitis B and C, which cause inflammation of the liver, and human immunodeficiency virus (HIV), the virus responsible for acquired immunodeficiency syndrome (AIDS). From 1979 to 1985, thousands of people with hemophilia worldwide were infected with hepatitis and HIV viruses from using contaminated blood products.

Reducing Risk

In the 1980s, methods using heat and chemicals were developed that inactivated viruses such as HIV, making it safer to use plasma and plasma precipitates to treat hemophilia. These methods are still used today. Another way to reduce the risk of catching diseases from blood products is to use a man-made substance that would encourage blood to clot. For example, in 1977, Professor Pier Mannucci of the University of Milan in Italy discovered that a compound called desmopressin could be used to treat mild cases of hemophilia type A and von Willebrand's disease. Desmopressin is a synthetic, or man-made, hormone, a compound that affects the way that other compounds or organs in the body behave. Desmopressin increases the release of factor VIII and von Willebrand factor, which in some cases of mild hemophilia and von Willebrand's is enough to address the problem.

DNA and Hemophilia

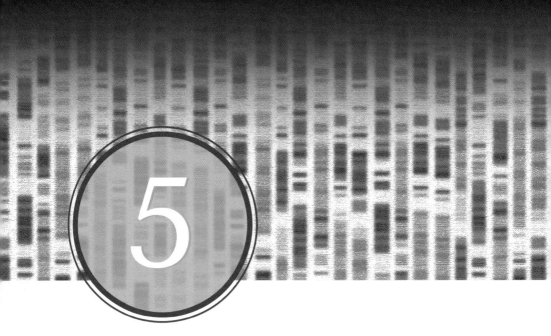

The fact that traits could be passed from parents to children was recognized from earliest times. However, it wasn't until the twentieth century that the mechanisms by which this occurred were fully understood. In the first half of the twentieth century, scientists established that DNA was the carrier of genetic information. DNA contains four nucleotide bases: adenine (A), thymine (T), cytosine (C), and guanine (G). Genes consist of different combinations of these four bases. In 1953, English scientists James Watson and Francis Crick, along with Maurice Wilkins and Rosalind Franklin, discovered the three-dimensional structure of DNA. They figured out that DNA is a double helix, or two strands twisted around each other in a way

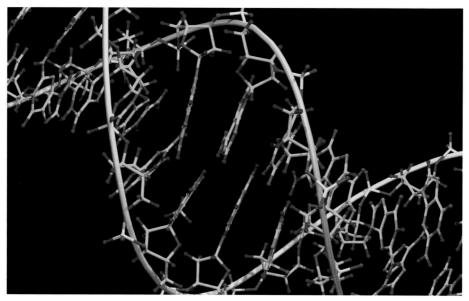

This photo shows a computer model of DNA. Each of the two strands contains a base *(blue-red)* attached to an outer sugar-phosphate backbone *(yellow)*. The four types of bases link up in complementary pairs. Cytosine attaches to guanine and adenine attaches to thymine.

that resembles a spiral staircase. Watson later went on to become head of the Human Genome Project, whose mission was to map the location of all the genes on human chromosomes.

Sequencing the Human Genome

In order to identify the cause of genetic diseases and treat them, it was first necessary to establish the location of each gene, the exact arrangement of bases in it, and the protein it codes for. This was made possible by the invention of techniques for

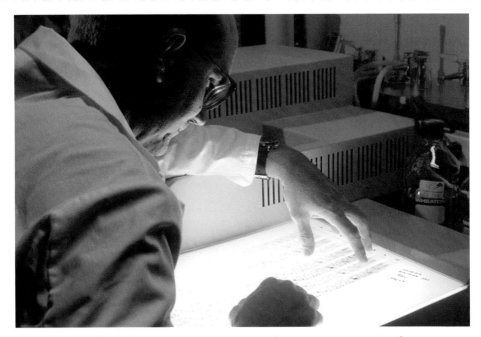

A process called electrophoresis is used to separate DNA fragments by size. This process results in an autoradiogram, like the one being examined here. The autoradiogram shows a "ladder" of bands. Each band represents a single DNA base. Each human gene has a unique sequence of DNA bases.

sequencing genes. When scientists sequence genes, they use chemicals to separate the gene into its bases and identify the order in which they occur. In 1977, the first process for this was developed by Fred Sanger while working at the University of Newcastle in England.

In the mid-1990s, automated methods of sequencing DNA were invented, which made the process of gene sequencing much faster. The Human Genome Project started in the United States in 1990. Its goal was to sequence the entire human genome by 2005. In 1998, a competing project was started by Dr. J. Craig Venter and the Applera Corporation. Their company, called Celera Genomics, had the goal of sequencing the entire human genome within three years. They met their goal, sequencing the entire genome by June 2000.

In addition to locating and sequencing genes, a second set of techniques was necessary to treat a genetic disease like hemophilia. The goal of these techniques would be to change a "bad" gene into a "good" gene. In the 1970s, two discoveries took place that made such a transformation possible. In 1970, a type of protein called a restriction enzyme was discovered. A restriction enzyme can cut strands of DNA at specific points, allowing it to be used to "cut out" a bad gene or a portion of it. Then in 1973, American scientists Stanley N. Cohen and Herbert W. Boyer developed methods of inserting new DNA into a strand of DNA that has been cut by a restriction enzyme. This new combination of genetic material is called recombinant DNA.

Finding the Factor VIII Gene

In 1984, the gene for factor VIII was discovered by Jane Gitschier and colleagues at the Genentech company in San Francisco, California. Identification of the gene for factor VIII made possible genetic-based treatments for hemophilia, such as infusions of what are known as recombinant clotting factors. In 1992, Wyeth, a pharmaceutical company, succeeded in creating the first recombinant version of clotting factor VIII. This factor, called rAHF (recombinant antihemophilic factor) is used for the treatment of hemophilia type A. It is produced by inserting the gene for clotting factor VIII into animal cells, such as those from Chinese hamster ovaries. The cells then multiply and begin to produce the clotting factor, which is collected. The factor produced in this fashion is the same, biochemically, as that extracted from human plasma. However, because it does not come from human blood, it is less likely

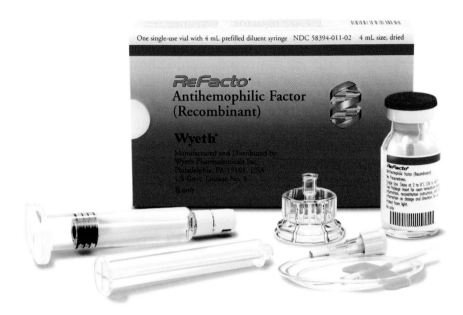

One single-use vial with 4 mL prefilled diluent syringe   NDC 58394-011-02   4 mL size, dried

ReFacto
Antihemophilic Factor
(Recombinant)

Wyeth

Manufactured and Distributed by:
Wyeth Pharmaceuticals Inc.
Philadelphia, PA 19101, USA
US Govt. License No. 5
R only

Pictured above are the contents of a package of ReFacto, a recombinant form of factor VIII produced by Wyeth Pharmaceuticals. It comes in a single-dose kit that includes a syringe prefilled with the solution needed to dilute it.

to contain impurities such as viruses that might infect those who receive it.

In February 1993, a second recombinant factor VIII product, Kogenate, was developed by another pharmaceutical company, Miles Inc. of Elkhart, Indiana. Kogenate is currently available from Bayer Healthcare, which acquired Miles. One concern with some of the earlier recombinant factors such as Kogenate is that they use albumin, a human protein, in their manufacture. This can result in contamination of viruses and may cause an allergic reaction in some people. In response to such concerns, the Genetics Institute and Wyeth developed a recombinant factor IX, called

BeneFIX, in 1997. This product is used to treat hemophilia type B. It is produced without the use of plasma or albumin and is, therefore, less likely to cause adverse reactions or infection. In 2002, Wyeth began selling ReFacto, an albumin-free form of recombinant factor VIII. Bayer Healthcare now also offers an albumin-free version of Kogenate, called Kogenate FS.

There is also new hope for patients who develop antibodies to factors VIII or IX. Recombinant factor XIIa is being developed as a treatment for patients who have inhibitory antibodies to these factors.

There are drawbacks to these types of products, however. They remain active for only a short time, so they must be given frequently. Also, they are expensive. Recombinant factor treatments usually cost more than nonrecombinant treatments. Recombinant DNA treatment for a person with severe hemophilia can cost $100,000 or more per year.

Although all these approaches are a step forward in treatment, they still rely upon replacement of the missing clotting factor. They do not actually cure the underlying problem that causes hemophilia. The next chapter looks at some new technologies aimed at curing hemophilia.

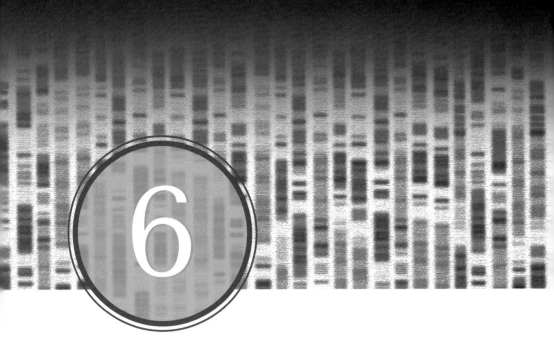

What the Future Holds

Genetic engineering, or altering the structure of genes, is key to the development of future treatment of hemophilia. The area of expertise that uses scientific techniques to change the structure and chemistry of genes at their most basic level is known as molecular medicine. Hemophilia, because it is a genetic disorder, lends itself particularly well to such an approach.

 ## Making Better Clotting Factors

One future genetic engineering method is aimed at modifying the recombinant clotting factors discussed in the last chapter. One such approach aims to delete the part of the factor

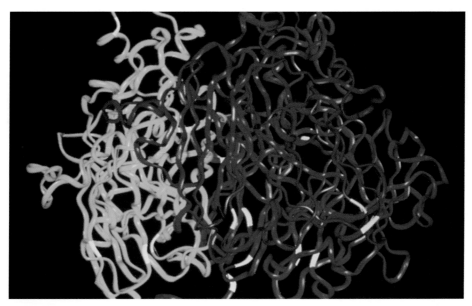

This photo shows a computer model of the factor VIII protein. It is a very large and complex molecule composed of three parts called domains *(shown in red, blue, and green)*. The unique shape and composition of the molecule determines how it interacts with other molecules in the body.

that allows it to be broken down, or degraded, in the body. If the factor is not degraded, it will remain active in the body for longer periods of time.

Another area being explored is how to reduce the effect of inhibitory antibodies in patients who receive the clotting factors. Research is presently going on that is directed at creating a hybrid factor VIII molecule that is produced by combining human and pig gene sequences. It is hoped that the majority of inhibitory antibodies will bind to one portion of the hybrid factor, leaving the other free to act. In the future, we are likely to see the development of other recombinant clotting factors that contain fewer of those sequences that produce inhibitors in patients receiving them. This should improve the effectiveness and reduce the cost of treating people who have an inhibitory response to the clotting factors currently available.

Replacing a Defective Gene

The ultimate solution to the problem of dealing with hemophilia would be to find a cure. One way being explored to do this is gene therapy. In this approach, a defective gene is replaced with a fully functioning one, which will result in the patient producing his or her own clotting factors. Hemophilia is an excellent candidate for treatment with gene therapy because the disease, unlike many other genetic diseases, is caused by a single defective gene. Theoretically, if there were a way to replace the defective gene with one that functions normally, the problem would be solved.

Identification of the gene for factor VIII and development of recombinant DNA techniques have made it theoretically possible to treat a person with classic hemophilia by replacing the defective gene for factor VIII with one that functions correctly. There are still problems that must be worked out with this approach, however. One difficulty is that the gene for factor VIII is very large and complex compared to other genes.

In the most common approach to gene therapy, genes that produce a given protein, in this case factor VIII or IX, are inserted into a deactivated virus. This type of virus has been altered so that it cannot cause disease. Adenoviruses are commonly used as carriers, or vectors, for new genes. When the viruses carrying the good gene are injected into a patient's bloodstream, they attach to the patient's cells and insert the good gene. This causes the patient's cells to produce the desired protein.

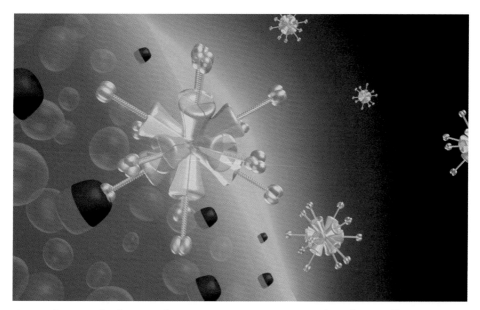

Capsules made from adenoviruses are seen in the above illustration. Inside the capsules are the genes used to replace those that are defective. The viruses' natural ability to penetrate cell walls and place genes in cells makes them an excellent delivery mechanism.

This technology has shown promise in experimental trials with animals. For example, scientists have had success replacing a nonfunctioning gene for clotting factor IX with a working one in dogs at the Children's Hospital of Philadelphia and in mice and dogs at the Stanford University School of Medicine. In early trials with human beings, some improvement in the production of clotting factors was initially seen, but the improvements were not permanent. In addition, although no ill effects were observed in these patients, some researchers have raised concerns about the use of viruses in human gene therapy. They fear that the viruses might spread to other people or be transmitted to the children of people treated with them. Despite the lack of success so far,

A CONTROVERSIAL THERAPY

The term "germ line" refers to egg and sperm cells. Soon after an egg cell and sperm cell combine, they begin to divide into two new cells. These cells then divide to form four cells, which divide to form eight cells, and so on until an entire embryo is formed, eventually becoming a fully formed human.

Since every cell in the human body comes from an original combined sperm and egg cell, every one of the body's cells contains the same genes as in these original germ cells. When the fully grown human produces its own sperm or egg cells, these cells, too, will only contain genes found in the original sperm or egg cells. Thus if one of the genes in the original sperm or egg cell is changed, that altered gene could be passed on to future generations. In experiments performed using mice, scientists have found this to be true. This is an important difference between germ-line gene therapy and the type of gene therapy used to treat people after they are born. In the latter type of therapy, genes in cells in the patient's body are changed, but the patient's sperm or egg cells still carry the patient's original genetic information.

Although germ-line gene therapy could possibly prevent the problem of defective or missing clotting factors in hemophilia, it is a controversial procedure. Some people feel that it is not right to alter the genetic makeup of germ cells. They argue that when the germ cells are changed it changes the genes of the patient and also the genes of any future generations, possibly with unexpected results. Because of this controversy, most research being done on gene therapy is aimed at treating patients after they are born.

and despite the controversy, researchers working on gene therapy are still hopeful that an effective method will be discovered in the future.

On the positive side, it is not necessary for gene therapy to be 100 percent effective, completely curing hemophilia. If treatment could simply increase the amount of clotting factor produced, this could be a life-changing difference. For instance, if a person who produces only 1 percent of the normal amount of clotting factor could produce 5 percent, moving him or her from severe to mild hemophilia, that person could live with much less fear of bleeding problems. He or she would only need extra clotting factor in special situations, such as when undergoing surgery.

Nonviral Gene Replacement

In response to concerns about using viruses in gene therapy, some researchers have been investigating other vehicles for gene transfer. One promising approach to treating hemophilia relies on implanting new cells. In this method, cells called fibroblasts are implanted directly into a patient. Fibroblasts are a type of cell found in connective tissue and are capable of secreting proteins. Normally, in the body they secrete collagen, which is used in the connective tissue that supports muscles, such as tendons and ligaments. In the case of hemophilia, the fibroblasts are genetically engineered to produce factor VIII instead.

In one trial, investigators inserted sequences for the factor VIII gene into fibroblasts removed from six patients. The fibroblasts were multiplied in the laboratory, and then the engineered cells were implanted back into the patients. The patients were monitored for a year, and the majority of patients showed an increase in the production of factor VIII and a

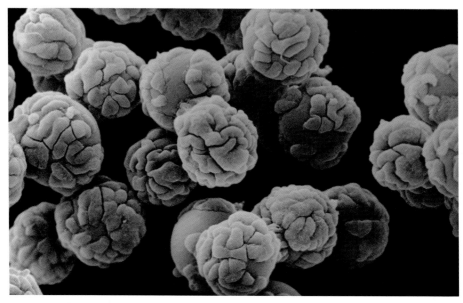

Human fibroblasts may be used to treat hemophilia in the future. After genes for the production of factor VIII are inserted into human fibroblasts, the fibroblasts that successfully secrete factor VIII are selected. The fibroblasts are then implanted into the wall of the patient's abdomen.

decrease in bleeding. Interestingly, no inhibitors of factor VIII were produced within the patient's own body.

Scientists in China are experimenting with using skin cells as a mechanism for gene transfer. The clotting factor gene is inserted into skin cells taken from a patient with hemophilia. The cells are then grown in cultures in the laboratory. When enough cells have been grown, the cells are implanted under the skin of the patient. The Chinese scientists did this successfully with two patients. The treatment resulted in patients who had been producing 2 percent of the amount of normal clotting factor producing 4 percent (a significant improvement in clotting level for someone with hemophilia). Because this treatment uses the patient's own skin cells, it could reduce the response of inhibitors to the clotting factor.

Fixing a Broken Gene

Another approach being investigated by researchers involves fixing a gene so that it produces the protein it should be producing. Sometimes hemophilia, as well as many other genetic disorders, results from a mutation in a gene's sequence that stops the gene from making a protein, such as a clotting factor. A new drug being developed by PTC Therapeutics, known as PTC124, addresses this problem.

According to PTC Therapeutics, PTC124 is taken by mouth, so it does not require injection with a needle. It targets nonsense mutations on genes. Nonsense mutations are changes at a single point of the genetic code that prematurely halt the process by which a gene produces a protein. This results in a shortened, nonfunctional protein (such as that for one of the clotting factors). PTC124 allows the cellular machinery to bypass the nonsense mutation and continue the protein-producing process, restoring the production of full-length, functional proteins.

In 2005, PTC124 was approved by the U.S. Food and Drug Administration (FDA) for use in clinical trials for treating muscular dystrophy and cystic fibrosis. Among the other diseases under consideration for possible treatment is hemophilia. The advantage of PTC124 treatment is that it is a generalized treatment. It could work on a wide variety of genetic disorders that result from the same common type of mutation— a sequence of DNA bases on a gene telling it to stop functioning before the protein the gene codes for is produced. This is much simpler and more widely applicable

TCGATTCTGAACATGATACGTACTGGTCCACTAGAACTGAACTCGAGAGGTACTA

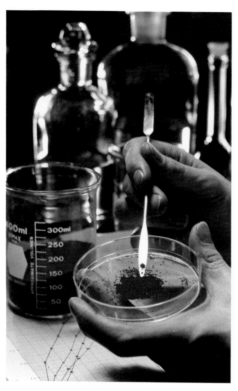

A chemist examines micros-phere capsules used to deliver medication. Manufacturing microspheres with a uniform size allows for controlled release of medication, making it more effective. Molecules enclosed in microspheres often remain active longer than those delivered directly into the bloodstream.

than gene therapies that require correcting a mutation on the gene for one specific variety of one particular disease. Not only would it help people with a variety of genetic diseases, but it also would probably be available much sooner than gene therapies. Not all genetic diseases are caused by premature stop mutations, so PTC124 would not help everyone, but it could improve the lives of many.

Futuristic Devices

Another innovative approach is being investigated by Dr. Harvey Pollard and his colleagues at the Uniformed Services University School of Medicine in Bethesda, Maryland. They are working on a device that will be implanted in the abdomen of a patient and continually convert the inactive form of factor VII into its active form, VIIa. Factor VIIa causes the coagulation cascade to happen and eliminates the need to use either clotting factor derived from blood or genetically engineered factor VIII or IX.

Another experimental approach to increase the amount of clotting factor in blood involves the use of microspheres. These are hollow spheres less than 1/10,000 inch in diameter. These tiny spheres can carry genes into cells or proteins in the bloodstream. Experiments with rats have shown that genes carried by microspheres that are fed to the animals can find their way into cells. This opens up the possibility of their use as a nonviral delivery method for gene therapy. In addition, the researchers demonstrated that proteins can be released into the bloodstream from the microspheres. This creates the possibility of delivering clotting factor in an oral rather than injected form, which would certainly be welcomed by many.

An Optimistic Future

Advances in computer science are allowing researchers to model molecules and study how they behave. This provides scientists with the ability to screen for medications most likely to be effective. Now that the human genome has been sequenced, researchers are gaining a better understanding of the specific genes responsible for making proteins such as clotting factors. As we progress through the twenty-first century, we are likely to see these and other technologies mature and new approaches develop. Whether hemophilia can be cured remains to be seen, but it is likely that advances in science and technology will make it easier to live with the disease.

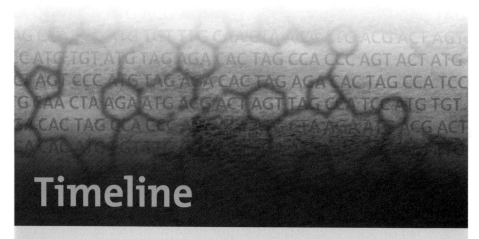

Timeline

1793
The first modern description of hemophilia is made by Dr. G. W. C. Consbruch of Germany.

1828
The term "hemophilia" is used in print for the first time by Friedrich Hopff, a German medical student.

1840
The first successful treatment of hemophilia by blood transfusion is performed by English physician Samuel Lane.

1853
Queen Victoria gives birth to a son, Leopold, who has hemophilia.

1904
Alexis, the son of Czar Nicholas II of Russia, is born with hemophilia.

1936
Plasma is first used to treat hemophilia.

1939
Kenneth Brinkhous at the University of North Carolina demonstrates that people with hemophilia lack factor VIII.

1955

American pathologists Kenneth Brinkhous, Robert Langdell, and Robert Wagner develop the first method of giving patients infusions of factor VIII.

1964

English physician R. G. Macfarlane identifies the coagulation cascade.

Mid-1960s

Judith Pool of Stanford University develops cryoprecipitates, simplifying the treatment of hemophilia.

1980s

Methods using heat and chemical processing are developed that inactivate viruses such as HIV, making the clotting factor derived from plasma safer to use.

1984

The gene for factor VIII is isolated and sequenced, making possible genetic-based treatments for hemophilia.

1992

Wyeth, a pharmaceutical company, succeeds in creating the first recombinant clotting factor.

1997

The Genetics Institute and Wyeth develop a human protein–free concentrate of recombinant factor IX, called BeneFIX, which can be used to treat hemophilia B.

2000s

Research begins into new ways of treating hemophilia, including nonviral gene therapy and implantable clotting factor delivery systems.

Glossary

antibody A chemical compound produced by the immune system that attaches to a foreign particle, marking it for destruction by immune system cells.

autoradiogram A type of photograph that is created when film is exposed to radiation, such as X-rays.

base In biochemistry, a segment of DNA. The four bases are adenine, cytosine, guanine, and thymine.

chromosome A long thread of DNA found in the nucleus of cells that consists of a series of genes.

classic hemophilia Another name for hemophilia type A.

coagulation cascade The process by which clotting factors work in series, with each affecting the next one to form a blood clot.

cryoprecipitate Solid material separated from plasma by a freezing and thawing process.

czar A king or emperor, usually referring to one of the former rulers of Russia.

deoxyribonucleic acid (DNA) The chemical compound that makes up chromosomes.

enzyme A substance that causes a chemical reaction in the body.

fibrin A chain of proteins that holds a blood clot in place.

fibroblast A type of protein-producing cell found in connective tissue.

fractionation The process in which a compound is separated into its component parts.

gene A segment of a chromosome that contains genetic information for a particular protein. A single gene or a combination of genes determine a trait, such as eye or hair color.

genome The entire collection of genes of an organism.

hormone A chemical in the body that affects the way that other compounds or organs in the body behave.

infusion A solution introduced into the body through a needle inserted into a vein.

meiosis The process that results in the formation of sperm and egg cells.

molecule A tiny particle consisting of two or more atoms held together by chemical bonds.

nucleotide The basic unit of DNA.

pathologist A physician who studies the causes of disease.

plasma The clear, yellowish fluid that remains when the solid blood cells are removed from blood.

platelets Cell fragments that clump together to form a blood clot.

prophylaxis Taking precautions to prevent a problem, such as a sickness, from occurring.

protein A type of substance found in all living things. Proteins are essential to the structure and function of cells.

rabbi A spiritual and religious leader of people of the Jewish faith.

recessive gene A gene that a child must inherit from each parent in order for the trait it codes to be expressed.

recombinant DNA A strand of DNA composed of DNA from different sources.

transfusion The transfer of blood from one person to another.

vector A vehicle used to deliver a gene in gene therapy.

virus A strand of DNA surrounded by a protective shell. A virus attaches to a cell and inserts its DNA into it, taking over the cell's internal components and producing more copies of itself. Eventually, the cell bursts, and the newly created virus particles attach to other cells in the body and repeat the process.

X-linked recessive A type of gene that occurs on the X chromosome. A male child who inherits a copy of the gene from his mother will have the trait the gene encodes for, but a female child will only have the trait if she inherits a copy from both her parents.

For More Information

Canadian Hemophilia Society
625 Avenue President Kennedy, Suite 505
Montreal, QU H3A 1K2
Canada
(800) 668-2686
Web site: http://www.hemophilia.ca

Hemophilia Association
4001 North 24th Street
Phoenix, AZ 85016
(888) 754-7017
Web site: http://www.hemophiliaz.org

Hemophilia Galaxy
Baxter Healthcare Corporation
One Baxter Parkway
Deerfield, IL 60015
(800) 423-2090
Web site: http://www.hemophiliagalaxy.com

Hemophilia Village
Wyeth Pharmaceuticals
5 Giralda Farms

Madison, NJ 07940
(888) 999-2349
Web site: http://www.hemophiliavillage.com

National Hemophilia Foundation
116 West 32nd Street, 11th Floor
New York, NY 10001
(212) 328-3700
Web site: http://www.hemophilia.org

World Federation of Hemophilia
1425 René Lévesque Boulevard W., Suite 1010
Montreal, QU H3G 1T7
Canada
(514) 875-7944
Web site: http://www.wfh.org

Web Sites

Due to the changing nature of Internet links, the Rosen
Publishing Group, Inc., has developed an online list of Web
sites related to the subject of this book. This site is updated
regularly. Please use this link to access the list:

http://www.rosenlinks.com/gdd/hemo

For Further Reading

Ballard, Carol. *Heart and Blood: Injury, Illness, and Health.* Chicago, IL: Heinemann, 2003.

Brynie, Faith Hickman. *Genetics and Human Health: A Journey Within.* Brookfield, CT: Millbrook Press, 1995.

Huegel, Kelly. *Young People and Chronic Illness.* Minneapolis, MN: Free Spirit, 1998.

LeVert, Suzanne. *Teens Face to Face with Chronic Illness.* Englewood Cliffs, NJ: Silver Burdett Press, 1993.

Naff, Clay Farris, ed. *Gene Therapy.* Farmington Hills, MI: Greenhaven, 2005.

Panno, Joseph. *Gene Therapy: Treating Disease by Repairing Genes.* New York, NY: Facts on File, 2004.

Potts, D. M., and W. T. W. Potts. *Queen Victoria's Gene: Haemophilia and the Royal Family.* Shroud, England: Sutton, 1999.

Resnik, Susan. *Blood Saga: Hemophilia, AIDS, and the Survival of a Community.* Berkeley, CA: University of California Press, 1999.

Sheen, Barbara, and Beverly Britton. *Hemophilia.* San Diego, CA: Lucent Books, 2003.

Willett, Edward. *Hemophilia.* Berkeley Heights, NJ: Enslow, 2001.

Bibliography

Aronova-Tiuntseva, Yelena, and Clyde Freeman Herreid. "Hemophilia: 'The Royal Disease.'" University at Buffalo, State University of New York. Retrieved June 7, 2005 (http://www.sciencecases.org/hemo/hemo.asp).

Bolton-Maggs, Paula H. B., and K. John Past. "Haemophilias A and B (Seminar)." *Lancet*, Vol. 361, No. 9371, May 24, 2003, pp. 1801–1809.

Bozdech, Marek, MD. "Hematology and Genetics: From Heredity to Molecular Biology." *Sonoma Medicine*, Vol. 56, No. 1, Winter 2005.

Burke, Michael G. "Gene Therapy for Hemophilia A." *Contemporary Pediatrics*, Vol. 18, No. 8, August 2001, p. 135.

Canadian Hemophilia Society. "All About Hemophilia: A Guide for Families." Retrieved June 1, 2005 (http://www.hemophilia.ca/en/13.1.php).

Coalition for Hemophilia. "Gene Therapy." *Factor Nine News*, Spring 1998. Retrieved July 7, 2005 (http://www.coalitionforhemophiliab.org/newsletters/1998-Q1.html).

Flieger, Ken. "Outlook Brighter for Youngsters with Hemophilia." *FDA Consumer*, July/August 1993.

Giangrande, P. L. F., Dr., "The History of Haemophilia."
Retrieved June 7, 2005 (http://www.medicine.ox.ac.uk/
ohc/history.htm).

Hemophilia Galaxy. "About Hemophilia." Retrieved July 7,
2005 (http://www.hemophiliagalaxy.com/patients/about).

Henahan, Sean. "Fido's Gene Therapy Success Bodes Well."
Access Excellence. Retrieved July 7, 2005 (http://www.
accessexcellence.org/WN/SUA12/hemophilia199.html).

Moore, Amy Slugg. "Apparatus Holds Promise for
Hemophiliacs." *RN*, Vol. 63, No. 6, June 2000, p. 104.

"New FDA Approvals." *Drug Utilization Review*, Vol. 19,
No. 9, September 2003, pp. 71–72.

Roth, David A., Nicholas E. Tawa Jr., Joanne M. O'Brien,
Douglas A. Treco, and Richard F. Selden. "Nonviral
Transfer of the Gene Encoding Coagulation Factor VIII in
Patients with Severe Hemophilia A." *New England Journal
of Medicine*, Vol. 344, No. 23, June 7, 2001, pp. 1735–1742.

Westphal, Sylvia Pagan. "Passing Stop Sign Cures Gene
Disease." *New Scientist*, Vol. 180, No. 2417, October 18,
2003, p. 16.

World Federation of Hemophilia. "History of Hemophilia."
Retrieved June 7, 2005 (http://www.wfh.org/
2/1/1_1_3_HistoryHemophilia.htm).

Wyeth Pharmaceuticals. "Wyeth Hemophilia History." Wyeth
Hemophilia Village. Retrieved June 7, 2005 (http://www.
hemophiliavillage.com/wyeth_history.asp).

Index

About the Author

Jeri Freedman has a BA from Harvard University and spent fifteen years working for companies in the biomedical and high-technology fields. She is the author of a number of other science books for Rosen Publishing, including *How Do We Know About Genetics and Heredity* and *Lymphoma: Current and Emerging Trends in Detection and Treatment*. She lives in Boston, Massachusetts.

Photo Credits

Cover top © Eye of Science/Photo Researchers, Inc.; cover inset, p. 1 © www.istockphoto.com/Rafal Zdeb; cover background images: © www.istockphoto.com/Arnold van Rooij (front right), © Jim Wehtie/Photodisc/PunchStock (front middle), © www.istockphoto.com (back middle, back right), © Lawrence Lawry/Photodisc/PunchStock (back left); pp. 7, 37 © Alfred Pasieka/Photo Researchers, Inc.; p. 9 © Steve Liss/Time & Life Pictures/Getty Images; p. 12 © Dennis Kunkel/Phototake; p. 15 © Wellcome Library, London; pp. 17, 20 © Hulton Archive/ Getty Images; pp. 19, 31 © Bettmann/Corbis; p. 22 © Custom Medical Stock Photo; p. 25 © Nat Farbman/Time & Life Pictures/Getty Images; p. 27 © Richard Haggerty Photography; p. 28 © John Watney/Photo Researchers, Inc.; p. 33 © St. Bartholomew's Hospital/Photo Researchers, Inc.; p. 34 © Linda Kahlbaugh/AP/Wide World Photos; p. 38 © Science Source; p. 40 courtesy of Wyeth Pharmaceuticals, Collegeville, PA; p. 43 © Francoise Sauze/Photo Researchers, Inc.; p. 45 © Kenneth Eward/ BioGrafx/Photo Researchers, Inc.; p. 48 © Dr. David Phillips/ Visuals Unlimited/Getty Images; p. 50 © Robert Isear/Photo Researchers.

Designer: Evelyn Horovicz; Editor: Brian Belval
Photo Researcher: Hillary Arnold